TITLE PAGE

Burantashi Aphrodisiac

Pausinystalia Yohimbe Sex Enhancer

Ebuka Ugboma

COPYRIGHT

DISCLAIMER

The information in this book is offered solely for educational reasons and is not meant to be a substitute for expert medical guidance, diagnosis, or care.

DEDICATION

This Book is dedicated to all Medical Workers all over the World.

TABLE OF CONTENTS

ABOUT THE AUTHOR

Ebuka Ugboma Esq FICMC, ACIArb UK, FMA, AGIS, PMP

LLB hons, BA hons, Dip Mus Ed, Pdip Bus Admin, PDip Estate Mgt, MBA, MSC Peace and conflict resolution.

Ebuka Ugboma has multiple degrees from different Universities across different fields; Arts, Law, Social Sciences and Humanities generally. He is a Chartered Arbitrator and Mediator, trained in the style and pattern of Chartered Institute Of Arbitrators UK.

Ebuka Ugboma has successfully published many books including Propensities And Habits For Success

Check out his books on Amazon:

https://www.amazon.com/Ebuka-Ugboma/e/B0B6HHVVW6

Email: garyugboma@gmail.com Phone: 2348033924157

WARNING

The information contained in this book is capable of turning you into a Bedroom Sex Bully. Proceed with caution.

INTRODUCTION

Burantashi Pausinystalia Yohimbe otherwise known as Yohimbe (Pausinystalia yohimbe) is an African evergreen tree. Its bark includes Yohimbe, a substance that has traditionally been considered as an aphrodisiac.

The Hausa Fulani tribe traditionally uses Burantashi Pausinystalia Yohimbe as a sex enhancer. Its literal meaning is "Penis rise up." Pausinystalia yohimbe is its botanical name. It is an aphrodisiac and a bitter stimulant. In Brazil, it is commonly referred to as "herba de coroa" and is used as an aphrodisiac and hallucinogenic stimulant.

Yohimbe bark is well-known for its ability to stimulate erection in men and reduce female arousal. It has also been used traditionally as an anti-depressant, and a treatment for various types of headaches, as well as to treat malaria. In Western medicine, Yohimbe is most often used as an aphrodisiac or male erectile dysfunction treatment.
Pharmacology

The active alkaloid Yohimbe found in the bark is structurally similar in structure to Dicyclomine, an anticholinergic agent, and acts on alpha and beta receptors. It binds directly to the alpha-adrenergic receptor (2), resulting in a direct stimulation of the sympathetic nervous system. Yohimbe also affects dopamine level and serotonin activity by forming a complex with monoamine oxidase, which prevents the breakdown of this neurotransmitter; this may be why it has been traditionally used for depression.

Shikimic acid and Yohimbe have been shown to be effective in increasing testosterone and sperm count.

The bark of the Pausinystalia yohimbe tree is used to manufacture a medicine known as Yohimbe. The active ingredients in the activated bark are generally referred to as Yohimbe or YH-7. However, this usage is misleading because the actual active ingredient present in the bark is often not present in its pure form. Yohimbe is a highly unstable molecule that breaks down into various products during manufacturing (e.g., part of the molecule disappears by hydrolysis). In addition, the drug may contain substances with similar mechanisms to Yohimbe.

Honokiol is another active ingredient found in Pausinystalia yohimbe. Honokiol (photo) is also a catecholamine agonist that acts on the sympathetic nervous system; however, honokiol is unique in that it also acts as an antagonist at various adrenergic receptors and prevents their stimulation of adrenaline release.

This is due to the fact that honokiol acts as an antagonist at alpha adrenergic receptors and beta adrenergic receptors. It is unclear how honokiol affects cortisol, but it may have a direct effect on steroid production.

The properties of Yohimbe and its effects on blood pressure, insulin, heart rate, and other mechanisms have been studied. In general, Yohimbe has stimulatory effects on central nervous system pathways which mediate various psychological functions; however, there are also peripheral effects of Yohimbe that affect sweat glands in the skin or gastrointestinal tract (irritation).

CHAPTER ONE

Uses And Benefits Of Pausinystalia Yohimbe

The bark of Pausinystalia yohimbe has been used for thousands of years in the treatment of various ailments. It has been used in Africa to treat the loss of sexual desire, which is often associated with past trauma; however, it is not clear what this means.

In Africa, Pausinystalia yohimbe bark has been used with some efficacy as a treatment for depression. In Cape Verde, Yohimbe has been used as a remedy for hyperkinesia and tremor in patients who have muscular dystrophy. The bark is also used as an anti-inflammatory agent to treat rheumatoid arthritis or osteoarthritis.

Pausinystalia yohimbe bark has also been used in Africa for the treatment of malaria. In fact, the most recent (2008) version of The Physicians' Desk Reference for Herbal Medicines states that Yohimbe is "potentiated by quinine and may potentiate quinine, resulting in cardiac arrhythmias".

CHAPTER TWO

The biology and scientific research behind Pausinystalia yohimbe

Pausinystalia yohimbe trees grow up to 30 m tall. They primarily grow in soil rich with calcium, magnesium and phosphorus. Yohimbe is also found in the bark of the Pausinystalia yohimbe tree and can be ingested or applied topically.

Yohimbe has been shown to have a glycoside structure. The Yohimbe molecule consists of three cyclic parts: the indole-3-propanoic acid, the 5-methoxy-2, 3 benzoxazolinone, and the 1-naphthylmethyl ester. It is chemically categorized as an indole alkaloid and is a bicyclic compound. Yohimbe is derived from an amino acid tryptophan and has both alpha agonists as well as beta blockers properties.

Yohimbe was first isolated in 1901, and the molecular formula was established to be $C_{20}H_{25}N_3O_2$. The structure of Yohimbe was not fully known until the 1960s when crystallographic studies were conducted. A nitrogen atom is present in one of the rings, which accounts for its indole alkaloid structure.

Yohimbe is most well known for its ability to increase libido. In fact, a recent study on mice revealed that Yohimbe increased sexual behavior probably by activating the excitatory neurotransmitters dopamine and noradrenaline in several parts of the mouse brain.

Although, Yohimbe has been shown through many studies to be effective in the treatment of erectile dysfunction, it is not a common medical treatment. In fact, Yohimbe is considered a schedule IV controlled substance by the Controlled Substances Act and can only be prescribed by a physician in cases where all other forms of treatment for erectile dysfunction have failed.

CHAPTER THREE

Pausinystalia yohimbe is also commonly used as a weight loss aid. A recent study on male mice revealed that Yohimbe can increase energy intake and decrease energy expenditure by acting as an appetite suppressant in insulin resistant mice, which are usually associated with obesity and diabetes. This study also found that Yohimbe could increase the weight loss of obese mice by increasing the efficiency of energy expenditure.

A study on the effects of Yohimbe on serotonin pathways was performed in rats. Rats were exposed to Yohimbe with a vehicle, and then placed in a chamber containing food. Then, they were observed over a period of time and were injected with an anti-serotonin drug after four days to see how their behavior changed. This experiment showed that Yohimbe increased serotonin concentrations, which plays an important role in the regulation of mood and anxiety levels through neural pathways.

This experiment also showed that Yohimbe can potentially help people with depression and anxiety disorders through the regulation of various serotonin pathways. This is significant because many anti-depression and anxiety drugs work by altering serotonin pathways in the brain.

Yohimbe has also been shown to decrease body weight, which may be a result of an increase in energy expenditure or an increase in caloric intake. A study on rats showed that Yohimbe increased food intake and decreased activity levels over a period of 14 days. It was suggested from this study that Yohimbe acts as an appetite suppressant.

Through the regulation of serotonin pathways, Yohimbe has been shown to have an effect on hormones as well. In particular, it acts as a beta blocker and an alpha agonist which is linked with altered estrogen levels, progesterone levels, and testosterone levels.

How Should Pausinystalia Yohimbe Be Manufactured?

Yohimbe is most commonly known for its effectiveness in the erectile dysfunction treatment market; however, it is often used in veterinary medicine and in South American traditions by people who are interested in enhancing their sexual lives. The products that are available from various laboratories are not necessarily pure Yohimbe; therefore there may be a risk of allergic reactions occurring when consuming these products.

Yohimbe can be extracted from the bark of the plant through a process called percolation chromatography. The key to this extraction process is to also include the decoction and boiling of the bark with water. The decoction and water extraction process can yield up to 4 grams of Yohimbe per 100 grams of bark. However, some laboratories may use a different method or may not use a decoct process at all.

What is the best way to consume Pausinystalia yohimbe?

In the past, Pausinystalia yohimbe was commonly consumed in barks, leaves and roots form by chewing or boiling. It is often used in its powder form as a nutritional supplement for boosting energy and increasing libido. Yohimbe has also been extracted from the bark of the Pausinystalia yohimbe tree to be used in a topical cream form for treating erectile dysfunction. Yohimbe can be ingested in some cases, but it has a bitter taste and is often used in combination with other herbs for a more pleasant taste. When taking the powder of the Pausinystalia yohimbe, it is best to take a single dose at a time and not to take more than two doses per day.

What Are Some Risks Associated With Pausinystalia Yohimbe?

Yohimbe is a drug that has been proven to be effective in the treatment of erectile dysfunction and in the weight loss market. It is also utilized by people who are interested in enhancing their sexual lives. In fact, studies have shown that the amount of Yohimbe that one can ingest without experiencing any effects would be comparable to taking one or two drinks of alcohol.

Side effects of Yohimbe, for those that are serious, can be problems with muscles, including the heart and blood vessels; severe anxiety and high blood pressure. However by taking Yohimbe in the appropriate dose, it does not cause any serious side effects such as anxiousness and high blood pressure.

CHAPTER FOUR

What Have Studies And Clinical Research Stated About Pausinystalia Yohimbe?

There has not been any major breakthrough in the medical or pharmacological world until the discovery of Yohimbe, which means that no one really knows a great deal about the effects of the substance. However, it is known to be an effective treatment for erectile dysfunction and is also used in weight loss treatments. Furthermore, studies are being conducted to evaluate the effectiveness of Yohimbe in treating various illnesses such as erectile dysfunction. It is also used by people who are interested in enhancing their sexual lives.

Why is Pausinystalia yohimbe used in the treatment of erectile dysfunction?

In the past, people thought that erectile dysfunction was caused by stress and overwork and that a person would go through a certain age where they would start to lose their capability to get an erection. However, studies have shown that erectile dysfunction has many different causes and usually begins at a young age; it is not something that occurs as we get older. Furthermore, there are no specific factors in a person's life that make them more prone to this disorder. Additionally, the causes of Erectile Dysfunction are varied and there has been no one cause identified for all forms of ED.

CHAPTER FIVE

BENEFITS

Depression Treatment

Dopamine is a chemical that helps the body and mind stay energetic and efficient. Furthermore, a lack of dopamine can cause mood swings, weariness, a lack of motivation, and even depression. Yohimbe has the ability to raise dopamine levels, which may be used to treat a variety of illnesses, including depression.

Aids In Weight Loss

Yohimbe has weight loss as one of its health benefits, therefore it is beneficial to persons who are overweight. It inhibits particular adrenoreceptors in the body while increasing norepinephrine levels. Norepinephrine inhibits fat mobilization while also breaking it down in specific challenging places of the body.

Reduces The Likelihood Of Hypertension

Yohimbe lowers the risk of hypertension by increasing blood flow in the body. When the body has good blood flow, it also protects several blood-related ailments such as hypertension, which you may read about in symptoms of high blood pressure. Furthermore, the disorder can set off other ailments in the body.

Improves Blood Circulation

As blood flow rises, it benefits general health. The increased blood flow means that the body's oxygen levels rise, which Yohimbe can help with. Yohimbe has traditionally been used as a vasodilator, which aids in the absorption of nutrients in the body.

Erectile Dysfunction Is Cured.

Yohimbe extract may help treat erectile dysfunction by increasing blood flow to the genitals. On the other side, it promotes fertility and increases desire. Some studies have shown this advantage, and it is one of the finest traditional uses of Yohimbe.

Aids Athlete Performance

Yohimbe helps people lose weight by increasing muscle mass and decreasing fatigue. Furthermore, it boosts energy, which helps athletes perform better. However, make sure you only take a small amount of it.

It Relieves Dry Mouth.

Yohimbe stimulates saliva production to keep the mouth moist or treats dry mouth. Dry mouth, also known as xerostomia, occurs when the salivary glands do not produce enough saliva. Furthermore, the illness could emerge as a side effect of treatment.

Yohimbe protects the heart from some disorders since it enhances blood flow in the body. Furthermore, it involves the removal of free radicals, which have been linked to heart disease.

Promotes The Healing Process

Increased blood flow leads to an increase in the healing process. Yohimbe stimulates the healing process, but in order to reap the maximum benefits, you need visit a doctor, especially if you have chronic ailments.

Cancer Prevention

Yohimbe's antioxidants remove free radicals, which leads to the reduction of cancer cells. Furthermore, some studies have shown that it can help with pain relief.

Yohimbe still has many health benefits, which you may learn about in uses and benefits of yohimbe. The benefits may work if you take it in moderation, because too much Yohimbe can have negative effects such as: Headache, Nausea, Dizziness, Anxiety, Failure of the kidneys, Paralysis, Hypertension, Tachycardia

CONCLUSION

Pausinystalia yohimbe raises your sexual performance with no adverse side effects. The herb is proven to be effective in the treatment of ED and PE. In addition, it can provide powerful health benefits that include boosting testosterone levels and increasing sexual self-confidence. Pausinystalia yohimbe also enhances intimacy for both you and your partner by eliminating premature ejaculation on the one hand, as well as prolonging their sexual activity on the other hand. While you can enjoy the benefits of Pausinystalia yohimbe, your lover will be able to feel satisfied and happy from your new-found sexual prowess and ability to satisfy her.

The medical benefits of Pausinystalia yohimbe also include being used to boost male libido, treat impotence, enhance sexual performance and treat premature ejaculation (PE).

Pausinystalia yohimbe enhances erectile response and endurance for both men and women.

Pausinystalia yohimbe is effective to treat erectile dysfunction and premature ejaculation with no harmful side effects. In addition, the herb helps to boost sexual performance and endurance for both genders. It also helps to increase your sexual self-confidence, satisfy yourself and your lover, increase intimacy, prolong intercourse and enhance sex drive.

The Hausa-Fulani tribe, which can be located in Nigeria and other parts of Africa, uses Burantashi Pausinystalia Yohimbe, a traditional sex enhancer or type of Viagra or manpower. Burantashi Pausinystalia Yohimbe is a pure natural product made from the violet tree's bark that helps to increase erection power while you are aroused and promotes better sexual health. Additionally, it encourages general wellbeing and good health. Burantashi Pausinystalia Yohimbe is a pure, natural herb that has long been prized for its unique characteristics.

When you are aroused, Burantashi Pausinystalia Yohimbe expands the erectile tissues of the Penis. When you get excited, the normal flow of blood fills these erectile tissues, which leads to an erection. grows and increases the size of these erectile tissues. This allows the tissues to contain more blood, which results in a much harder erection than before.

Burantashi Pausinystalia Yohimbe increases blood flow to the Penis, resulting in an erection that is significantly thicker, stronger, longer, and harder. Yes, the first and most obvious effects will be an increase in the firmness and power of your penis. You will also notice a decrease in premature ejaculation.

Does it have an impact on blood pressure?

Consult your doctor about any potential interactions Burantashi Pausinystalia Yohimbe may have if you are currently using a blood pressure medication. We firmly advise that you speak with your doctor before using Burantashi Pausinystalia Yohimbe if you have a medical history or are currently on any form of medicine.

Burantashi Pausinystalia Yohimbe advantages:

Put an end to Early Ejaculation, Increasing erection power, Keep your erection strong. Make your partner's sexual activity longer. Your sexual self-confidence should grow. Make your lover and yourself happy. Make more time for romantic pursuits.